HEATWAVES:

What to know about heatwaves, how to survive in heatwaves, and solutions to heatwaves

JASON A. ROBINSON

Table of Contents

Chapter One

Meaning of Heatwave

A heatwave is a lengthy period of excessively hot weather. A heatwave is a period of exceptionally hot weather, which may be accompanied by significant humidity, particularly in oceanic climate nations. While definitions vary, a heatwave is generally measured compared to the ordinary weather in the region and according to average temperatures for the season. Temperatures that individuals from a hotter environment consider usual might be labeled a heatwave in a colder place if they are outside the regular climatic trend for that area.

A heatwave is a protracted period of extremely high temperatures for a location. Though there is no standard definition in relation to how high. The temperatures have to exceed the historical averages for a certain location.

Causes of Heatwaves

Heatwave is a natural catastrophe yet a surge in it may be induced as a consequence of global warming. Heatwaves are created by a powerful high-pressure setting at about 10,000-25,000 ft. and refuse to move. This causes heated air to sink, the consequence is a dome of hot air that retains the heat near the ground and prevents cooling convection currents from producing clouds.

Heatwaves occur when there is trapped air that will feel like the interior of an oven! Usually, the cause is a high-pressure system that drives air downward. This force stops air near the ground from rising. The sinking air behaves like a cover, it traps warm ground air in position. Without rising air, there was no rain and there was nothing to keep the hot air from getting hotter.

Chapter Two

The Effects of Heatwaves

• On the Body

Heatwaves have several effects on the body ranging from skin to the blood to other body components. Some of the impacts include;

Sweating

It's your natural cooling system. Your body pumps sweat out onto the surface of your skin. As the air absorbs it, it takes heat away and cools you down. This works better in dry locations when humidity is low. You could feel extremely weary and even critically unwell if it doesn't work soon enough.

Dehydration

When it's excessively hot, you might sweat out too many liquids, along with critical minerals like salt and potassium. You may be thirsty and urinate less than normal, and your mouth and tongue can feel dry. You might even feel tired, lightheaded, and disoriented.

Heat exhaustion

It occurs in excessive heat when your body can't stay cool enough and sweats out too much water and salt. You become pallid and clammy, and your fever regularly soars beyond 100 degrees. You also may feel weary, weak, lightheaded, queasy, and have a headache. If you ignore it, it might develop into heatstroke, which is an emergency.

Confusion

You may find it tougher to focus and execute hard activities when things heat up. It's typically nothing to worry about, and you can repair it with a rest in a cool area and something to drink. But if you're already unwell from the heat and you get significantly confused about where you are or what you're doing, it might be a symptom of heatstroke, which requires rapid medical attention.

Heat rash

When you sweat so much that your sweat glands become clogged. When your pores can't get rid of it, you break out in little red pimples. It's more probable near your armpits, groin, neck, elbows, and beneath the breasts. Babies too may experience the same sort of response, particularly beneath their chin or in their crotch region.

Heatstroke

This is heat at its most deadly. You can't regulate your body temperature, which may go beyond 105 degrees. Your skin becomes heated and dry. You could feel confused or irritated and have a quick pulse, nausea, and a headache. If left untreated, it may induce seizures, and coma, and may be life-threatening.

Sunburn

Bare skin burns if it's in the sun too long. It may turn crimson, itchy, unpleasant, and heated to the touch. If severe, you might experience blisters, headaches, fever, and nausea. In the long term, sunburn raises the chance of getting skin cancer.

Heat edema

Heat might cause your fingers, toes, or ankles to swell and make your skin feel tight. It's not serious and normally goes away after you chill down and raise your legs. See your doctor if it causes discomfort, continues occurring, or doesn't get better.

Lower blood pressure

When you're hot, you sweat. That causes you to lose fluids and electrolytes. In addition, heat increases your blood vessel's dilation to enhance perspiration. Together, these substances may decrease your blood pressure, sometimes enough to make you dizzy or even pass out. It might be much worse if your heart doesn't pump regularly and isn't able to react to the additional demand.

Higher heart rate

When you are heated, your heart may beat quicker. It does so to pump more blood to your skin, where it may release some of that excess heat. As a consequence, other portions of your body may not receive enough blood. This might make you fatigued and sluggish, particularly if you're attempting to accomplish strenuous physical or mental work

Fainting

It's more common when you're new to a hot location, so take care to remain hydrated. Heat may dehydrate you and make it tougher for your brain to obtain adequate blood. That may make you dizzy and pass out. It could be worse if you stand for a long period or get up quickly. If you feel faint, lay down and lift your legs over your head. Go to a cool environment and consume fluids as quickly as possible.

Death

All symptoms of heatwaves, if not provided quick care may subsequently lead to the death of the affected individual.

- **On Agriculture**

Crop failure

Climate change is quite dangerous to agriculture. Higher temperatures eventually cause lower agricultural yields of desired crops while promoting the growth of weeds and pests. The probability of short-term crop failures and long-term output decreases rises with changes in precipitation patterns.

Heatwaves affect several aspects of crop growth and development, including soil moisture uptake, root and shoot development, photosynthesis, ventilation, plant water intake, and final yield. By accelerating evaporation, heatwaves compete with soil moisture, leaving practically little moisture for plants to absorb. Agriculture, forestry, and rangelands are particularly vulnerable to heatwaves because of the general environmental deterioration that is brought on by heatwaves.

- **On The Environment And Infrastructure**

Wildfire danger
A heatwave amid a drought can exacerbate bushfires and wildfires because it dries out the vegetation.

Infrastructure destruction

Heatwaves may cause power transformers to explode, water lines to break, and roads and highways to crumble and melt, all of which can result in fires. Additionally, heatwaves can harm railroads by buckling and kinking the rails, which can slow down traffic, cause delays, and even cause service to be suspended if the rails are too hazardous for trains to travel on.

Escalation of violence

People can become more aggressive when overheating. People often get more violent as they become more hostile.

Numerous power outages

Increased usage of air conditioning during heatwaves frequently results in electrical surges, which can cause power outages, aggravating the issue.

Economic productivity decline

People tend to become quickly exhausted during heatwaves as a result of stress, which slows down their rate of production over the long term.

Chapter Three

How to Survive in Heatwaves

Although there are several illnesses brought on by the heat, it is crucial to maintain your health while heatwaves are occurring. Here are a few tips for staying healthy while there are heatwaves.

Keep hydrated

Throughout the summer, being hydrated is crucial because it keeps your body functioning properly. The easiest way to do this is to consume more water. When you are away from home, you must always have a container of water with you for quick access. Alternatively, you may always buy bottled water.

Even if you don't feel thirsty, keep drinking water. During this time, when you tend to sweat a lot, it is crucial to replenish biological fluids lost by sweating.

Avoid consuming alcohol and caffeinated drinks

Consuming alcohol and caffeinated beverages affects the body and lowers its capacity to cope with the heat. Consuming this also leaves you craving more liquids. No matter how delicious or refreshing they are, they are not helping but injuring you. Take wate, reduce your alcohol and caffeine consumption since these beverages promote the process of dehydration.

Eat modest yet frequent meals to keep energy

Schedule your three meals into smaller ones to fight the natural fatigue that is produced by heat.

Also, keep away from heavy, hot meals. Meat and other heavy foods produce heat during preparation and digestion. Ensure that your meals include the required nutrients for maximum health. Include water-rich fruits such as watermelons, pineapples, berries, cucumber, and other similar fruits in your meals, plus veggies.

Avoid sex in high temperature

Avoid making love or having sex at times when the temperature is high, particularly around midday, since this activity exerts physical demands on you and elevates your heart rate.

Stay in the coolest parts of the house

If you have air conditioning, now is an excellent time to put it to use, particularly at night. It is most effective when other sources of heat are reduced, such as light bulbs. Make sure your house or workplace is well ventilated and open the windows when it is safe to do so.

Stay away from the sun

If possible, refrain from going outside when the weather is too hot. Prefer to go later in the day when the weather is cooler. As much as possible, stay away from the sun by staying inside or in shady locations. This is because, at high temperatures, dehydration sets up quickly.

Additionally, it raises the chances of acquiring skin cancer owing to the impact of harmful radiation from the sun. You may postpone outside activities during peak hours of sunshine, especially in the afternoons between 12 and 4pm. If you're working outdoors in the heat, stop and go inside to cool down, particularly if you feel lightheaded, disoriented, or faint.

Take baths as frequently as possible

If you begin to feel restless and you feel so hot, rush into the bathroom and take a shower. If you are not where you take a bath, damp a hand towel and put it behind your neck. You may also use it to massage your face. This helps to lower the body temperature.

Wear loose-fitting and light garments

Loose clothing permits airflow in between the fabric and your skin, enhancing aeration. This minimizes the heat created and the quantity of sweat produced. You should avoid black colors since they tend to absorb the sunlight leading you to feel hotter, and avoid synthetic materials that hold moisture and that generate extra heat. It is crucial to keep cool and for this reason, choose textiles that are light and would not absorb heat. Also avoid wearing heavy textiles, go with bolder hues of fabrics.

Avoid or reduce exercise

Regulate exercise and workout time and schedule. During exercise, the body generally responds with the heat. But these natural cooling mechanisms may fail if you're exposed to extreme temperatures for a long period. If you are new to exercising or you are unfit, be aware of what your body can manage and take pauses throughout your activity.

If you begin to feel pressure in your brain, or you are weak or dizzy, you need to stop and calm down. And if after some minutes you still feel dizzy, you may need to seek medical assistance. Also when you take long walks, at every opportunity you have, you should stop to cool yourself beneath a covered place. Avoid intense exertion if you can. This is because the more active you are, the more heat is created by your body.

Apply dusting powder or calamine lotion

As frequently as possible, use dusting powder or calamine lotion. This functions as a calming agent and helps chill the body.

Use sunscreen to protect your skin

The living wall works as a sunshade that helps decrease the ambient temperature in the courtyard and minimize heat absorption by the walls. When you move out in the sun, it is vital to put sunscreen on your skin to defend your skin from the sunlight. It helps lower the possibility of acquiring pigmentation, wrinkles, and skin cancer.

Use an umbrella, hat, and sunglasses as you go out

Whenever you go out in summer, it is necessary to protect yourself from exposure to the sunlight. The dangerous rays of the sun might cause your skin to dry, tan, pigmentation, and uneven. Use an umbrella, hat, and sunglasses anytime you venture out to protect your skin from damaging heatwaves.

Get an A/C or fan

Set your air conditioners to a lower setting and use curtains or blinds to keep glaring sunlight out. If A/C is not accessible, remain inside on the lowest level in a well-ventilated room with fans. Keep curtains and blinds closed. If you don't have air conditioners, set a tray or dish of ice in front of a fan and it'll assist to chill your space rapidly.

Get a backup generator

A backup home generator is the safest and most dependable choice! Power outages are prevalent during heatwaves because the requirement for A/C puts too much strain on the power infrastructure. A backup generator, however, automatically keeps the A/C running, the lights on, food and medication from rotting, and medical gadgets operational.

Pay attention to weather forecast

Be alert to weather predictions and the approaching temperature fluctuations. You should also follow weather reports and predictions to plan your outdoor activities whenever necessary..

Pay care to the old, the ill, children, and pets. Don't leave children or pets alone in hot vehicles. Keep your pets inside and ensure they have access to a cool spot and water. When you notice someone having a heat stroke, take them out of the heat and remove the outer clothes. Lay them down with the legs above their head, and fan them. If the individual has dry skin, administer moist compresses, then seek medical care.

Chapter Four

How to Solve Heatwaves Problems

There has been a surge in the incidence of heatwaves, which has called for immediate attention from people, organizations, and the government.

Irrigation system for agricultural

Irrigation is the artificial delivery of water to the land by different systems of tubes, pumps, and sprays. Irrigation will be crucial for keeping crops cool and for giving adequate moisture to fulfill their water demands. Crops may be kept cool by enhancing evapotranspiration. As liquid water evaporates heat is lost from the surfaces of leaves and soil and from the surrounding air, which cools the temperature of the crop.

Deforestation

When there is a spike in temperature or when the hot season is approaching, trees with no leaves, dry roots, and stems should be chopped down to prevent producing an increase in the case of Wildfires.

Afforestation

Afforestation is the formation of a forest or stand of trees in an area where there was no prior tree cover. Trees help counteract the greenhouse effect via the process of photosynthesis since they function as carbon sinks.

In other words, building new trees provides additional carbon dioxide-holding regions lowering the carbon dioxide in the ecosystem. The ultimate conclusion is the lessening of the impact of global warming. Government should support the planting of trees, and flowers in the garden.

Install cool roof and green roof

A green roof is a vegetative layer planted on a rooftop. Green roofs offer shade, remove heat from the air, and lower temperatures of the roof surface and surrounding air. Using green roofs in cities or other constructed areas with minimal vegetation might decrease the heat island effect, especially during the day.

Cool roofs are composed of highly reflecting and emissive materials that stay cooler than typical materials at peak temperatures. Both cool and green roofs give advantages of reduced surface and air temperatures, and less energy consumption.

Artificial rain

Cloud seeding is a sort of weather manipulation that tries to influence the quantity of precipitation that falls from clouds by releasing chemicals into the air that function as cloud condensation or ice nuclei, which alter the microphysical processes inside the cloud.

Paint roof white

Black roofs are said to draw a lot of heat, roofs should be painted white to prevent the rate of heat in the home.

Let wind blow

To decrease heatwaves, High Rise buildings, and constructions that restrict the free blowing of air should be avoided as much as possible. When there is free circulation of air, the dwellings will be properly ventilated. It is also crucial to remember that; in the case of heatwaves, constructing the higher layer homes grows hotter owing to its nearer to the sun.

Use appliances with less energy

Home appliances that consume little energy must be used in the house to reduce electricity spikes and power grid failure to avoid an outage of electricity.

Reduction in global warming

Greenhouse gas emissions must reach zero as soon as feasible. All nations need to transition their economies away from fossil fuels as quickly as feasible. Fossil fuels include coal, oil, and gas - and the more they are mined and consumed, the worse global warming will grow. Changing our primary energy sources to clean and renewable energy is the greatest strategy to quit using fossil fuels.

9 798845 630483